The Dieter's Guide To Weight Loss After Sex

by Richard Smith

Workman Publishing
New York

Acknowledgement

To those who let me watch.

Library of Congress Cataloging in Publication Data

Smith, Richard.
    The dieter's guide to weight loss after sex.

    Continues the author's The dieter's guide to weight loss during sex.
    1. Sex—Anecdotes, facetiae, satire, etc. 2. Reducing—Anecdotes, facetiae,
satire, etc. I. Title.
PN6231.S54S56   1980   818'.5407   79-56531
ISBN 0-89480-081-7 (pbk.)

Jacket design: Paul Hanson

Workman Publishing
1 West 39 Street
New York, New York 10018

Manufactured in the United States of America
10 9 8 7 6 5 4 3 2 1

Contents

I. Recuperating from Sex

II. Rolling Over and Going to Sleep

III. Sleep

IV. Why We Wake Up

V. Life

VI. Love

VII. Even More Sex

How much weight do we lose after sex? Although current litera-
ture* exhaustively details the calories burned during foreplay,
intercourse and orgasm (real, faked and a blend), information
concerning weight loss between sexual encounters has, until
now, been sparse.

To be sure, for most people, sex—and its immediate spin-
off, more sex — appear to be a favorite form of dieting, more
popular than, say, skipping meals or having a tooth capped. Many
dieters, in fact, have gone so far as to assume that weight loss
without sexual activity (or a reasonable facsimile) is impossible.
Others, wishing to keep trim but unable to obtain adequate sex,
in desperation turn to golf, running and mineral water. Yet, as we
shall see in the following pages, weight loss does not have to
cease just because sexual activity has. Surprisingly enough, it is
often *after* sexual activity, commencing with the vital recupera-
tion period (expressing gratitude, getting the pulse rate down,
scolding a merciless nymphomaniac) and continuing until the next
sexual encounter that the real weight loss takes place.

In some cases, just talking a reluctant partner into leaving
will burn almost fifty-four calories—more if it's not your apartment. Showering with a partner who stays, on the other hand,
can burn over sixty-two calories, especially if you dry each other
with a mop. If you're both on vacation, the post-coital effort of
removing each other's snorkel outfit may shed nearly seven
ounces.

Those who choose not to recuperate from sex, preferring
instead to roll over and go to sleep, will discover that sleeping, a
seemingly passive activity, burns an enormous number of calories, especially if it's done quickly. And weight loss potential
increases for sleepers who toss and turn or occasionally suffer
the torments of a meatloaf-induced nightmare.

The weight loss process continues as we go about the
normal, mundane aspects of life, such as falling in love or kicking a
vending machine. Stifling yawns during a business meeting, for
instance, can erase the calories in that morning's martini; Christ-
mas shopping for an aunt who has nothing will burn off a large

*See *The Dieter's Guide to Weight Loss During Sex.*

glass of wine. Smiling at a co-worker's ugly baby pictures can shed up to forty calories and, possibly most slimming of all, summoning the courage to open a mechanic's repair bill may drain the body of all of its calories.

The Dieter's Guide to Weight Loss After Sex also covers many high-intensity activities which, though they consume numerous calories, require no special equipment. For the first time ever, the serious dieter has, at his or her fingertips, information such as the caloric contrast between falling in love in Paris and falling in love in a K-Mart, along with the calories burned while sustaining a relationship or breaking one up, including dividing possessions, interfaith divorce (where applicable) and finding a new partner.

All in all, there are nearly 1,400 answers to the question most asked by serious dieters: "Is there life after sex?"

And finally, despite its title, *The Dieter's Guide to Weight Loss After Sex* does not suggest that sex as a means of weight loss should be eliminated. We have, therefore, in addition to a chapter on the latest in sexual research, also included calorie counts for what might be termed sex under extraordinary circumstances—while suffering from heartburn, while working in the office (with and without holding calls) and when helping your partner with calculus—foreplay while solving equations, for instance.

For a better idea of how we burn calories, see the following examples.

Table of Caloric Consumption

It takes nearly 2,400 calories a day to power a typical human being. What activities will increase this figure?

Activity	Calories burned
Trout fishing	63
Selecting new wallpaper	58
Commuting	84
Examining poultry	77
Gossiping	31

Sex

Intercourse	90
Lasting a long time	61
Moaning	16
Begging for more	8
Getting it	153
Orgasm: one	28
two	46
five	90
none	4
not giving up	120

After sex

Calling a truce	7
Rolling over	11
And going to sleep	2

I. Recuperating from Sex

For many people, it's after sex, during the crucial rehabilitation period, that the real weight loss begins, the theory being that going through the motions of life is more difficult than going through the motions of sex, which requires less coordination. There is also the gravitational reality— standing up takes more effort than lying down, especially if you're numb.

In this chapter we show that the restorative process means more than just regaining your land legs. It's everything—how you feel, how your partner feels and when to try again.

Stopping

Activity	Calories burned
After orgasm	1
Just before orgasm	245

When Should Sex Terminate?

Why stop at all? Why call a halt to an activity so pleasurable that it is often compared with Southern cooking. The answers to this question can be divided into three categories: lack of time, lack of energy and lack of interest. More specific reasons for ending sexual activity are listed below, not necessarily in order of importance or occurrence.

- Coming up for air
- Nothing left to try
- Nothing left (seed spilled)
- Desire for coffee and a bran muffin exceeds desire for partner
- Spouse waiting to be buzzed in
- Major shift in thought pattern—from erotic fantasies to this year's tax bite.
- Partner asking "Which way to the bar?"
- Partner suddenly responding to beeper
- Fourteen-inch bedsore
- Health precaution: one partner fermenting

Catching Your Breath

Too winded to smile? Mysteriously painful toes? Of primary importance is eliminating the symptoms of all-out sex: rapid pulse rate, laborious breathing and shaky metabolism. Instead of stopping abruptly, however, enjoy a leisurely warm-down period,* allowing the body to remain at rest until you can once again stand on your own two knees.

Activity	Calories burned
Panting	9
Gasping	14
Wheezing	19
Audible heartbeat	26
Very audible heartbeat (*neighbors banging on the wall*)	45
Receiving oxygen	18
Giving off helium	60
Putting head between your knees (*to prevent fainting*)	11
Putting head between partner's knees	17
Whiffing smelling salts	24

*Skip leisurely warm-down period if partner's spouse suddenly comes home.

Cooling Down

Of course you're tired—you've been pushing—get the pulse rate down and avoid cramps by tapering off gradually with a few gentle exercises.

Activity	Calories burned
Stopping the clock.	4
Releasing each other (de-entwining)	8
If you're stuck together	55
Fanning yourself	10
Fanning your partner	17
Slowly walking a quarter of a mile	25
Slowly crawling a quarter of a mile	41
On a deep-pile carpet	70
Whispering sweet nothings	9
If partner hard of hearing	22

Calling In Sick

Activity	Calories burned
The morning after	3
The night before	25
In order to continue sexual activity	21
In order to continue recuperating	6
If you have a guilty conscience	37
While moaning	52
Trying to sound ill	11
If sex was marvelous	85
Calling in well	2

Was It Worth It?

Among conscientious dieters, pleasure is much less important than weight loss. The question, "Was it good for you?" will almost always take second place to, "Did I lose weight?"

Activity	Calories burned
Measuring waistline 7	
With a yardstick 164	

How Soon After Sex Is It Safe To:

Start the car	5 minutes
Scold your partner	20 seconds
Start a rumor	3 hours
Thread a needle	20 to 30 minutes, depending on when your hands stop shaking
Undergo surgery	10 minutes
Operate dangerous machinery *(a dessert spoon, for instance)*	1 hour
Visit Japan	2 days
Take your leave	45 minutes
Criticize partner's performance	1 day
Assess partner's performance	1 minute

Remove prophylactic
    Regular
    Twist-off
	
	3 minutes
	30 minutes

Try again	15 minutes to several days, according to erectile recovery time

Staying the Night

Should it be a sleep-over date? With married couples, this question seldom arises. But if you're just getting acquainted, there are several factors to be considered. Sure, you can borrow a toothbrush (or use the handle if you're squeamish), share the slippers and use Windex on your contact lenses. You're even comfortable about requesting a glass of water for your teeth. Before making a final decision, however, consider the following:

Activity	Calories burned
Staying the night if	
Invited	3
Not invited	224
Sex left you fulfilled	3
Sex left you unfulfilled	67
Sex left you totally fulfilled but you want your teddy bear.	95
Partner is already snoring	31
And it's only 3:30 in the afternoon	73
Nothing in the refrigerator for breakfast	25
Except club soda and salmon croquettes	47
Partner's children keep asking who you are	100
Your children keep asking who you are	418

Expressing Gratitude

How do you tell your partner that it was fabulous, that not only the earth, but the entire solar system moved and you'd be more than happy to honor his or her credit card?

Activity	Calories burned
Massage	
Fingertips	26
Tongue	100
Back rub	18
Back tickle	12
Making lemonade from scratch	14
Brushing partner's teeth	7
Pedicure	17
Ticker tape parade	1,924
Installing marquee over bed	353
Putting partner's name in lights	141

The Sensual Bath

Activity	Calories burned
Alone	25
With your turtle	68
If you're just good friends	30
With your partner	42
Washing each other's back	55
Washing each other's chest	182
If tub double-parked	241

Making Sure There's a Next Time

Did you perform poorly? Do you now feel uncomfortable? There's no reason not to have a second chance. Simply dispel the tension by explaining what happened. Your partner will understand.

Explanations	Calories burned
Too much alcohol	7
Not enough	50
That it was your first time	28
That it was your first time with a partner	77
Conflicting astrological signs	32
Biorhythms out of sync	23
Too dark to follow the sex manual	38
Couldn't figure out what to do with hands	59
Poor shelf life	64

Encouraging Partner to Leave

Activity	Calories burned
If it's your apartment	45
If it's your partner's apartment	367

Trying Again

Why not? Even if the bed has been made and you've both gotten dressed, that's no reason not to explore the frontiers of exhaustion. Those who find the re-seduction process difficult, who can't recall the order in which things are supposed to happen, may find it easier to start with last things first.

Activity	Calories burned
Orgasm first	78
Then intercourse	
Without erection	283
Without insertion	350
Then premature ejaculation	392
Trying to feel aroused	411
Lust	500
Preparing the bedroom	120
Bringing in the garbage	45

How Do You Know When You're Ready for More Sex?

Activity	Calories burned
Bedsores healing nicely.	20

Closing Lines

Last impressions count. So decide what's most important—total honesty or just getting out of there without too much of a fuss.

Activity	Calories burned
All utterances	
If true	6
If false	45

Examples
> "We don't take Master Charge."
> "Call me."
> "I'll call you sometime."
> "I'll call you when I get back."
> "Please send me that recipe."
> "I'm listed."
> "Don't worry, I'm not listed."
> "Can we still be friends?"
> "Don't bother, I can let myself out."
> "Frankly, Murray, I don't give a damn."

II. Rolling Over and Going to Sleep

Should you choose not to recuperate, you may skip the previous chapter, yet still enjoy several weight loss alternatives. Succumbing to sleep directly after sex is no cause for alarm since, as many sleep researchers point out, post-coital repose may be either a healthy reaction to fatigue or, simply, a reaction. In many cases, this sleep state is only temporary and the sleeping partner, if pestered diplomatically, may awaken and grant a rematch.

Unfortunately, the partner still awake may feel rejected, especially if, instead of sweet nothings, the sleeper murmurs "Wake me at seven," and then goes off to dreamland.

Rolling Over and Going to Sleep

Activity	Calories burned
After orgasm	2
After arousal	28
Before orgasm	37
Just before orgasm	71
During orgasm	150
While still at the movies	9
Rolling over and feigning sleep *(to escape an excessively vigorous partner)*	45
Rolling over and hitting the wall	28
Rolling over and hitting the wet spot	365
Skidding	10
Sliding over and going to sleep	18

Reasons for Rolling Over and Going to Sleep

Activity	Calories burned
Heredity	50
Whipped cream all gone	18
Partner did it first	22
Socks caught fire	33
Partner doing nails	28
Elbows gave out	66
Lack of staying power	10
Lack of going power	9
Partner's gold chain knocked you unconscious	40
Too much Aramis	15
Partner recalled	98
Test tube full	10

Reactions of Partner Still Awake

Activity	Calories burned
Relief	14
Insomnia	26
Staring at ceiling	8
Squinting at ceiling	11
Displaced sexual energy	
Biting pillow	15
Attempting mouth-to-mouth resuscitation	42
Drum practice	60
Shaking martinis	28
Orgasm, self-inflicted	42
Closing the Murphy bed	14
With partner still in it	92

Reaction of Partner Still Asleep

Activity	Calories burned
Zzzzzzzzzzzzzzzzzz..............................	unlimited

III. Sleep

In the course of a lifetime the average American, unless bitten by a tsetse fly, will sleep nearly 178,850 hours (though seldom all at once) and the lazy American nearly 225,000 hours. But just what is sleep? Previously thought to be passive resistance to standing upright, researchers now tell us that sleep is a natural, normal response to growing sleepy. Once asleep, they point out, the sleeper sleeps until he is finished; he then wakes up and stretches. Too much sleep, however, can lead to prolonged lying down which, if too prolonged, eventually leads to death, and the sleeper —except in rare instances—will not require a hot breakfast. It is to prevent this that the body, during a sound and delicious sleep, mobilizes its defenses and makes us wake up to go to the bathroom.

Sleep, of course, is not always caused by sex. Nearly 96 million Americans go to sleep each night without sex, simply because they are either sleepy or have nothing better to do.

Fortunately, for those interested in weight loss, sleep is not so passive an activity as one might imagine. It has, in fact, more calorie-burning potential* than many waking-hour activities. Just lying on your back and finding a comfortable position for your head, one in which your nose isn't stabbing the canopy, can burn up to twenty-two calories. Confirmed late sleepers will find, to their delight, that the agony of getting up at 6:30 A.M. on a cold, rainy Monday morning to punch in by 8:00 A.M. is calorically equivalent to carrying a papoose to Honduras. And coping with an erratic electric blanket that can also fry potatoes may burn off ninety-one calories plus vaporize your toes. (It should also be noted that the speed at which one sleeps greatly influences calories burned.)

*Especially during that magical period between sleepy and asleep, a state known as "sleepish."

Varieties of Sleep

When is sleep not sleep? To be considered official, the act of sleep must be performed in one continuous motion, with a beginning (growing drowsy), a middle (asleep, possible snoring) and an end (waking up). Anything else, though there may be a noticeable suspension of consciousness, cannot properly be called "sleep," but rather a form of inertia in which the eyelids either close or droop. To date, researchers have classified over six hundred forms of inertia, the most common of which are listed below:

Activity	**Calories burned**

Dozing 26
>Lightweight sleep—perfect for those too tired to sleep. It can occur with surprising suddenness, during a sermon, while on guard duty or after an especially restful orgasm. Symptoms include violent fluttering of the eyelids and uncontrollable nodding of the head.

Snoozing. 19
>A sneakier, less sincere form of dozing. Hand is often placed over the eyes, suggesting that the snoozer is deep in thought. Indispensable for jurors in a humid courtroom, economics students and when attending message plays written by a rich relative.

Napping 30
>Much deeper than snoozing, but not as deep as authentic sleep. For maximum efficiency, a nap should take place on a couch or Barcalounger just before dinner or right afterward with a newspaper or large sun hat over napper's face. Nap aids include a hot water bottle and a blanket knitted by any blood relative such as mommy.

Featherweight napping and one of the
shallowest versions of sleep known to
science. Catnappers almost never dream or
receive an in-depth visit from the Sandman.
The catnap is handiest when sitting out
traffic jams, working in an all-night gas
station or waiting for the *Robert E. Lee*.

First cousin to the nap. Doesn't count unless
taken during daylight hours, preferably after
lunch in the back room of a store or at your desk.

The polar opposite of a dead faint.

May occur without warning. A common
reaction to enthusiastic sex between
partners in poor condition. May also happen
at a dinner party in response to the
conversational abilities of the person to your
left, in which case you pitch face forward into
your glass of Chablis.

Often mistaken for fitful slumber and the
least gracious form of repose. Usually
precipitated either by a meatloaf with
bauxite, organic Snickers bars or a neighbor
showing slides of her trip to the A&P.

A serious form of hibernation.

A microcoma and hitherto unknown particle
of sleep. Occurs during vital waiting period
between end of televised campaign speech
and its translation by news analysts into English.

Preparing for Sleep

Activity	Calories burned
Filling the water bed	33
Yawning	2
Brushing teeth	8
Vacuuming teddy bear	11
Checking under bed for burglars	5
Finding one	263
Turning down covers	3
Turning down partner	
Headache	6
Rough day at the office	9
Wrong day of the week	12
Staying awake to watch "Tonight Show"	
Carson the host	23
Carson not the host	100
Listening to "Rock-a-Bye Baby"	6
Drinking warm milk	15
Directly from goat	75
Leaving a wake-up call	10
Leaving a tuck-in call	25
Saying prayers	5
Just mumbling them	37

Trying to Fall Asleep

Activity	Calories burned

Under ideal circumstances 3

Under less than ideal circumstances
    Faucet dripping................................ 20
        On your face 99
    Lumpy bed 10
    Outerspring mattress........................... 31
    Truck backfiring 14
    Partner backfiring............................. 26
    Feet longer than blanket 57
    Home fries repeating 36
    Elusive itch.................................. 42
    Partner practicing Rotary Club speech 147

Finding a Comfortable Position

Falling Asleep

Activity	Calories burned
All at once	6
Section by section	125

Section by section includes eyelids growing heavy, breathing slowed and sleep-inducing thoughts such as, "toes, go to sleep," "nighty-night, ankles," "pleasant dreams, knees," etc.

Remaining Asleep

Once asleep, weight loss goes on, through the effort of what scientists and some laymen accurately describe as "staying asleep."

Activity	Calories burned
For light sleeper	56
For heavy sleeper	5
For really heavy sleeper . . . . *(over 400 pounds)*	51

Note: Wear a nightcap. Ninety percent of lost sleep seeps out through the head.

Positions

Fetal 27
     Popular not only with insecure adults, but
     the favorite position of most unborn babies.

Scrunched up 38
     An advanced version of fetal. Preferred by
     those wearing tight pajamas. Sleeping in this
     position takes up less than one square foot of
     surface area. If there are enough blankets on
     the bed, the sleeper will never again be
     heard from.

At attention 45
     Arms and legs rigid, face pointing skyward.
     Widely used by credit managers.

At peace 15
     The ultimate position, with sleeper on top,
     bed on bottom. The sleep of fools and those
     with a clear conscience.

Restless 81
     Sleeper on bottom, bed on top.

Spoon 23
     Allows the woman to take full advantage of
     male body heat. Man faces severe
     reprimand should he move away.

Upright 56
     For waiting in post office lines. And surviving
     dull parties. Not recommended during a tax
     audit.

Interruptions to Sound Sleep

Activity	Calories burned
Going over potholes	35
Sequined nightshirt	20
If sequins on the inside	44
Nightcap made of wood	16
Sleep mask overheating	19
Decorator sheets with raised design	50
Guilty conscience	166
Visions of sugarplums dancing in head	23
Clumsy tooth fairy	30
Boisterous visit from the Sandman	38
Partner demanding a glass of water	75
Partner in heat	42
Tinkle emergency	25

Sleep Disorders

Activity	Calories burned
Insomnia	
Tossing and turning	30
Staring up at ceiling	10
Staring down at pillow	15
Both at once	50
Pacing: back and forth	28
up and down	70
Worrying about not sleeping	100
Sleepwalking	40
Sleepjogging	78
Talking in sleep	14
Talking too much in sleep	345

Snoring

Usually occurs when the nose, like a sink, backs up. Some psychologists suggest that snoring represents either an unconscious need for attention or hostility toward one's partner. Snoring may also indicate that, for the time being, sexual activity is over.

Activity	Calories burned
For snorer	
Regular	7
Rattling fixtures	19
Unsettling plaster	45

For listener	115

Silencing snorer	
Plunger	10
Clothespin	7
Paper clip	3
Pastry tube	18
Noose	185

Dreamland

Why do dreams consume so many calories? The answer, postulates author J.T. Velour (*I Dream of Jeannie with the Light Brown Pantsuit.* Vienna, 1979), is that the sleeper is doing three things at once: lying still, sleeping *and* dreaming. Calories burned are determined by where the dream originates—id, ego, superego or upset stomach. In addition, interpreting the dream without a licensed gypsy can increase the calories burned by 15 percent.

Activity	Calories burned

Source of dream

Id (located at base of head) 41
    Produces dreams of a vigorously sensual
    nature. Lots of mysterious symbols, many of
    them sexual—moaning bananas, wilting
    cigars, curvaceous chickens and rowing to
    Germany in a kayak.

Ego (somewhat higher, about eye level) 30
    Dreams from here a bit tamer, many
    acceptable as family fare. Lots of wish-
    fulfillment and frustration. You are the mayor
    of Disneyland but still can't board the rides
    for free. To make matters worse, you are
    constantly frisked by Mickey Mouse.

Superego (tippy-top of head) 23
    Short, more-to-the-point type dreams.
    Conflict is often the theme. Should I look for
    a job or go to the movies?—marry or
    continue having a rewarding sex life?

Upset stomach 78
    These dreams are rightly known as
    nightmares. They're often the result of a
    punitive expedition by a stomach filled with
    tainted Popsicles or a midnight snack of
    eggplant salad on Lorna Doones.

Waking Up

A time when many people who are ordinarily quite genial find themselves cursing the day they were born—hostile to everything except an opportunity for more sleep.

Activity	Calories burned
Hearing alarm	24
Wondering where you are	15
Wondering if you are	60
Ignoring alarm	1
Silencing alarm	
Normal method	3
Violent method	18
Feeling sorry for yourself	15
Cramming in extra moments of sleep	32
While someone is shaking your shoulder	47
Telling shaker to # &%('*	20
Promising to get up in five minutes	4
Getting up in five minutes	104

Getting Out of Bed

For a professional late sleeper, the effort of unfastening oneself from the bed, especially if it's magnetic, burns more calories than sawing wood. On a cold morning, just coaxing a toe—any toe—to peep out from under the quilt can burn off last night's pie and ice cream. Making that supreme effort and finally standing upright (both feet on floor, no part of body making contact with bed) can compensate for eight ounces of marmalade. Indeed, it is not uncommon for those with extreme difficulty arising to carry a security mattress wherever they go.

Activity	Calories burned
Getting out of bed	78
Seriously considering calling in dead	150
Attempting to walk	63
Losing traction	12
Attempting to march.	85
Giving up	2
Just letting your fingers do the walking	103

Hangover

The picture changes completely if the joy of arising is marred by a hangover, especially one that maims. The victim will frequently find the effort of throwing back the covers too much for one person and may have to do it section by section.

Activity	Calories burned
Misery, general	43

Headache	27
If splitting	54

Focusing eyes on any object smaller than the wall	30

The shakes	61

Severe caloric expenditure just trying to hold hand still enough to shave. Many find it easier and safer to hold razor still and move the face.

Throbbing	19

Eating	86

Effort here is not eating itself so much as holding down what has already been eaten. Sufferer advised to temporarily refrain from kasha and anchovy paste.

Attempting sex	250
If partner also has hangover	500

IV. Why We Wake Up

In this chapter, we offer the latest research on a previously neglected source of weight loss, for it is only in the last few years that weight loss scholars have accorded the bathroom the serious consideration warranted by the often magisterial activities of its occupants.

Recent studies show that for many, the bathroom is more like a workshop, even a chapel, in which visitors pass the time in a productive and highly contemplative manner—solving problems, reading, doing the crossword puzzle, reconciling a stubborn checkbook and, in general, getting their lives in order.

Americans, in fact, spend a good deal of their disposable and even indisposable time either in the bathroom or in desperate search of one, especially after partaking of ethnic delicacies in a strange part of town. (It is not unusual for a dieter, upon finally finding an acceptable comfort station, to expend nearly twenty calories begging for the key. Witness one family who drove the entire length of the New York State Thruway before finding a clean rest room, and then burning, collectively, sixty-eight calories pleading with a sadistic service station attendant to unlock it.)

Internal Distress

"Most accidents occur within fifty feet of an unsanitary taco stand."

Few realize the marvelous slimming opportunities provided by a sudden attack of intestinal discomfort, the result, perhaps, of poorly bred sausage, barbecue sauce with a high atomic weight or capturing first prize in a German chili-eating contest. Until you find relief, exercising restraint will burn a torrent of calories, especially if you're cursed with a low pain threshold.

Activity	Calories burned

Exerting self-control and putting on a happy face (although knuckles whitening) after ingesting

Chicken salad on whole wheat	19
Bean curd	48
Black coffee and a Lucky Strike	85
Bolivian water	62
Guacamole: regular	45
industrial strength	98
Black beans and rice: American (sissy) style	37
Spanish (macho) style	100
Authentic Szechuan food	141
All-Bran in suspension of warm prune juice	350

Internal Combustion

Activity	Calories burned
Regularity	14
Too much regularity *(six visits before a job interview, for instance)*	45
Extreme regularity *(six visits during a job interview)*	60
Irregularity	29
Worrying about it	250
Grimacing	8
Squirming	12
Straining	23
If lumbago acting up	35
Sweating and shivering	7
Breaking wind	
In half	7
In quarters	14
Being creative	
Genteel "blip"	3
Regular "phooooph"	12
Enormous "whoppeeeeeeee"	25
Gale-force "kraaaaaaaaaaaaaaaaaaa" *(often caused by bellicose corn relish)*	38

Doing Two Things at Once

For busy people, the bathroom is a perfect place to catch up on one's reading. All that is needed is proper lighting and no unusual surprises.

Reading	Calories burned
Periodicals: *Readers' Digest*	7
Sunday *New York Times*	250
Paperback: Nixon's memoirs	28
Hardback: Kissinger's memoirs	25½
Reading between the lines	
Kissinger's memoirs	195
Nixon's memoirs	300
Computer printout	18
Toilet paper	10
Someone's palm	28
Doing crossword puzzle	15
Polishing off a coloring book	30

Interruptions and Distractions

Few events are more annoying and possibly traumatic than having one's privacy disturbed, especially unnecessarily. The greater the imposition, the more calories burned.

Activity	Calories burned
Camel sobbing	45
Insistent spouse	11
Persistent Avon lady	22½
Persistent insurance salesman	23
Outhouse repossessed	29
With you in it	87
Civil disorder	50
Phone ringing	18
Resisting urge to answer	32
Answering	
Hopping to phone	41
Catching breath	15
Wrong number	65
Returning to point of origin	27
Restoring tranquillity	10
Kids screaming to get in	100

The Perfect Houseguest

The problem of discretion while visiting someone's home is often highlighted when using the bathroom, especially when the door is wafer thin.

Activity	Calories burned
Locking door. 3	
No lock 28	
Holding foot against door. 32	
If commode is eight feet away 90	
Trying to be silent 22	
If you've eaten too much herring salad. 122	
Attempting loud coughs during crucial moments 18	
If your timing is poor 75	
Whistling a merry tune 15	
Singing "On the Road to Mandalay". 19	
In a booming baritone 26	
If you're a woman 40	
Singing "You Light Up My Life". 12	
While doubled over 50	

Vanishing Without a Trace

Activity	Calories burned
Opening window	6

If no window	30
And it's hot and humid	41
And somebody is waiting to get in	50

Turning on exhaust fan	3
Exhaust fan surrenders	45

Last-ditch efforts

Glade	10
Brazilian cigar	14
Applying roll-on deodorant to walls	35

Acting nonchalant as you walk out	51

Feeling responsible for person's death	100

The Amenities

We asked a panel of wine experts for their considered opinion on things less haughty than Bordeaux but just as glorious.

V. Life

Is it possible to burn calories just by *being*? Does simply standing there, wondering whether to ask for a date, help to shed pounds? Experts who have grappled with this question assure us that the mental energy needed to make even a marginally interesting life work provides an excellent basis for an ongoing program of weight control.

Again, as in previous chapters, we must caution against the fallacy of associating weight loss only with highly suggestive activities such as sex, Ping-Pong and shopping. Trying to make sense of your new toaster warranty, for example, can burn more calories than eight minutes of foreplay. Firmly refusing a Hare Krishna solicitor at an airport can knock off a quick two ounces and being polite to odious in-laws consumes the caloric equivalent of skating to Rio.

In this chapter we will see how millions of dieters, just by participating in this thing called "life," and standing up straight, can drastically improve their appearance.

Looking Out for Number 1

Activity	Calories burned
Hoarding canned goods	34
Wearing garlic	7
Wearing protection	9
Crossing yourself	4
Doubling-crossing yourself	8

Driving defensively
Automobile	14
Shopping cart	20

Activity	Calories burned
Wearing gloves in public lavatories	7
Making sure he really had a vasectomy	10
Before he's removed his clothes	48
Maintaining an unlisted number	2
Maintaining an unlisted face	31

Getting In Touch with Inner Self*

You are you and I am me
You did your thing
I did your thing
No wonder we are no longer friends
SWAMI BOTSWANA VERANDA, MARCH 10, 2152 B.C.

The constant struggle for self-awareness is the pathway to resolving the conflict between who we are, who we would like to be and who our parents would like us to be.

Activity	Calories burned
Meditation	14
If assisted by controlled substance	2
If assisted by uncontrolled mantra	54
Voodoo	29
Open-head surgery	310
Being at one with your surroundings	36
In a museum	41
In a Woolworth's	97
Nonjudgmental volleyball	88
Actually touching your soul	60
Getting your hand wet	160

*Not always a good idea.

Self-Improvement

Activity	Calories burned
Getting reborn	989
Using original womb	15,256

Coping with reality	
Yours	17
Reality's	381

Whipping self into shape	
Small whip	16
Large whip	40
Cool Whip	81

Getting act together	158
Dismantling act	7

Keeping nose to grindstone	23
While it's turning	289

Leaving home at	
Age eight	10
Age twenty-four	245
Age forty-one	5,000

Self-Assertion

Have you ever accepted a collect call from a person selling light bulbs? Afraid to say no to a toll collector? Stuck with more Amway products than you'll ever need? For those who are timid, but determined, the agony of self-assertion presents constant opportunities for weight loss. The more fainthearted, the more weight lost.

Activity	Calories burned
Sounding horn in a hospital zone	11
Asking neighbors to return your lawn mower	17
While they're using it.	63
Insisting on a refund	
At the supermarket.	15
From your hairdresser	57
From a used car dealer named Arnie	138
Asking butcher to grind meat in front of you.	29
Refusing a fourth helping of mashed potatoes	
In a restaurant.	5
At your mother's house.	40
At your mother-in-law's	90
Demanding a raise	60
That you don't deserve.	97
Refusing to have sex	
If date spent less than $5 on dinner	2
If date spent more than $40 on dinner	36

Self-Acceptance

Who am I? Along with a mirror and an up-to-date ID, accepting who you are can be a crucial step toward achieving full potential, be it a promotion into the mail room or finally learning to cut your own hair.

Accepting that you are:	Calories burned
You	325
Someone else	15
Always in the mood for sex	23
Even with your spouse	75
Losing your hair	31
But only twelve years old	90
Never going to hate rich desserts	52
A lover of trashy novels	60
Only four feet, six inches tall	89
But not Napoleon	124
A slave of passion	7
A slave	100
Never going to get into shape	31
Never going to leave North Dakota	56
But multi-orgasmic	2

Self-Rejection

Activity	Calories burned
Lying about your age.	15
To your parents.	62

Self-Destruction

Activity	Calories burned
Blowing your brains out	8
With a fan	265
Licking postage stamps	3
With additives	5
With nonkosher glue	7
Serving warm beer to a longshoreman	15
Mixing scotch with borscht	37
Biting off more than you can chew	19
During sex	81

Nerve

(Burns even more calories than courage.)

Activity	Calories burned
Picking up a "ten"	30
By the scruff of the neck	66
Buying irregulars	18
Giving them as gifts.	49
Cash bar at your daughter's wedding.	75
Standing up to a delicatessen waiter	
Insisting on lean pastrami	54
And a clean fork.	78
Asking exhausted spouse for sex	40
For even more sex	68
If exhausted spouse not yours.	100

Frustration

(One of the perils of being away from home.)

Activity	Calories burned
Visiting public rest room	8
If coin-operated	12
But you have nothing smaller than a fiver.	97
Squeezing under door	74
Somebody already there	145
Patiently waiting	11
If mission urgent	30
Remaining jovial	44
Clenching teeth.	27
Breaking into a sweat	18
Breaking into a dance	70

Panic

Activity	Calories burned
"Out of Order" sign	200

Joy

Activity	Calories burned
Feeling your oats	26
Feeling someone else's oats	150

Guilt

When it comes to weight loss, the classic causes of guilt — excessive tax deductions, not calling parents on their anniversary and shoplifting are calorically insignificant. Sexual guilt,* on the other hand, a form of unconstructive energy, can burn off calories at an astounding rate, depending on the individual's sensitivity.

Activity	Calories burned
Constantly fantasizing about sex	12
Especially during foreplay	26
Especially during lasagna	54
Sex when you should be working	35
Working when you should be having sex	½
Going AWOL at an orgy	20
Saying yes	44
And hating yourself in the morning	51
Saying no	44
And hating yourself that night	51
Instant orgasm	1
Having more orgasms than your partner	3
Intercourse	16
If there was penetration	58

* It is puzzling that guilt is so often caused by sex, a no-fault activity.

Surprise

The greater your astonishment, the more calories burned. The only exception is getting hit by a car which, though startling, does not burn too many calories.

Activity	Calories burned
Waking up married	108
Finding money	
On the street	17
In your wallet	44
Receiving a Dear John letter	64
From your mother	91
Finding out that masturbation really does cause insanity	500
Receiving an obscene phone call	31
If you like it	47
Receiving an obscene house call	89
Getting caught in bed	
With spouse	11
By spouse	1,158

Shock

Activity	Calories burned
10 volts... 18
110 volts... 87

Rejection

Activity	Calories burned

By

Humiliation

Activity	Calories burned

Applauding at the wrong moment
    At a concert 16
    At a meal. 24
    At a funeral 60

Frontal nudity
    During sex 7
    During an inspection 85

Falling off your partner 52

Falling off the bed 97

Premature ejaculation. 48
Begging for another chance. 62

Premature ejaculation during self-abuse 8
Begging yourself for another chance 77

Getting caught with your pants down 80

73

Anger

Experts tell us that the body sheds calories according to the degree of pique. Just getting hot under the collar, for instance, burns thirty-four calories, whereas flying into a rage, especially if your feet leave the ground, consumes nearly ninety calories.

Activity	Calories burned
Getting stuck with the dinner check	27
For the fifth time that week	49
With the same people	76
Getting a tie for Christmas	17
Getting a Thai for Christmas	85
Partner doing a number on you	
Number 1	100
Number 2	500
Partner regards you as a sex object	42
But does nothing about it	63
Partner can only climax if holding teddy bear	36
Teddy bear wearing flea collar	90

Expressing Anger

Activity	Calories burned
Flying off the handle	25
Climbing back on	48
Changing kitty litter	11
With kitty still in it	36
Crushing beer can with bare hands	20
Crushing beer bottle with bare hands	127
Serving dinner guests	
Warm Tang	11
Uninspected chopped meat	18
Out-of-season chopped meat	52

Self-Maintenance

Activity	Calories burned

At the dentist
Root canal............................156
  Without novocaine...................2,518
Listening to dentist's jokes.......................156
  Without novocaine...................2,518

At the doctor
Checkup by kindly family doctor...................56
Checkup by hostile proctologist.................1,000

At the psychiatrist
Lying on couch..............................3
  Face down..............................50
Interpreting dreams: yours......................28
    your psychiatrist's............100
Five-tissue session..........................45
Twenty-tissue session........................90

At the hospital
Getting hospital food...........................65
Keeping it down..............................149

Various Maladies

Which afflictions are most dietetic? To be sure, passive annoyances such as bunions and liver spots are of little consequence in the battle to lose weight. Other problems are a different story.

Activity	Calories burned
Pain and itching	11
Resisting urge to scratch	28
Scratching	20
In public	59
Shrinking hemorrhoids through	
Ointment	22
Surgery	75
Dry cleaning	92
Prayer	108
Coughs due to	
Colds	16
Chicken bones	248
Headache	
Taking two aspirin	4
Cranial by-pass operation	395
Possession by	
Demons	27
Heartburn	56
Calamari	81
Repossession by	
Finance company	147
Mother country	500

Compulsive Behavior

That irresistible impulse to again check the front door lock, recite the alphabet each morning and fold each sock — all may seem irrational but they burn calories.

Activity	Calories burned
Activating taps with your elbows in public washrooms	24
Placing paper on the seat	14
Even if you're there only to wash your hands	98
Making bed	11
Just before going to sleep	39
Thumb sucking	
Yours	6
Your boss's	42
Calling parents	
Every night	15
Every time you have sex	30
Every time you don't have sex	67

VI. Love

Next to sex, falling in love and the ensuing benefits—a meaning-ful relationship, living together and buying a dog—provide the greatest number of calorie-burning opportunities. For those fortunate enough to have a meaningful relationship that also includes sex, the weight loss possibilities become enormous and you may actually need dietary supplements such as cake and veal tablets.

A meaningless relationship, on the other hand, can also be calorically beneficial as long as you both compensate for having little in common by stepping up sexual activity.

For those who have both a meaningful relationship (in which you grow) and a meaningless relationship (in which you shrink) there is little to worry about and you may, with no adverse effect, partake of rich desserts.

Relationships

Activity	Calories burned
In which you act like a caring, sharing human being	567
In which you act like yourself.	23
Getting into a relationship	11
Getting out of a relationship.	394
Living without someone you can't live without.	406
Living with someone you can't live without	750

What's in a Name?

Pay attention to your new partner's name—it could be a promise of things to come. Making a relationship work with a Harold, for instance, will doubtless be easier than with a Sergio. The same holds true for women. Susans and Marys are invariably easier companions than, say, Muffins or Sydneys. See additional examples below.

Name	Calories burned by partner
Ronald, Paul, Charles	17
Sluggo, Biff, Cheech	85
Murray, Roger, Eugene	34
Haskell, Phineas, Spike	55
Gaylord, Hugh, Orville	47
Chauncey, Rudolf, Abner	77
Shirley, Bertha, Lorraine	35
Evelyn, Elizabeth, Virginia	20
Heather, Twyla, Melody	45
Muffie, Buffie, Fluffie, Scruffie	66
Wendy, Debbie, Barbie	27
Adrianne, Raquel, Ursula	52
B.J.	138

Weight Loss Bonus #1

Activity	Calories burned
Falling for someone.	86
Falling in like	115
Falling in love	127
Falling head over heels in love	290
Sweeping partner off feet	212
With a broom	386
Falling at partner's feet	25
Falling on partner's feet.	80

Falling in Love

Do the seasons and our surroundings influence our love life? Experts, including travel agents, tell us yes—that the chances of falling in love in a romantic setting are greater than those in a mining town. A librarian, for instance, is more apt to feel romantic during a vacation in Paris than while collecting overdue fines in Denver.

Activity	Calories burned
In spring	
Paris	3
Rome	5
New York	8
Hong Kong	46
In fall	
New England	4
Canada	6
K-Mart	90
In winter	
A ski resort	10
Moscow	100
In summer	
The Caribbean	7
Khartoum	221

Love

Activity	Calories burned
Requited	50

Activity	Calories burned
Unrequited	357

Includes suffering, anxiety, obsession with love object, feelings of rejection and overeating.

Worshiping from afar
Three miles	41
Ten miles	118
Flirting through binoculars	220

Narcissistic love
Requited	44
Unrequited	303

Weight Gain Bonus #1

Falling in love can be calorically disastrous. At the onset of enchantment, both partners, overcome by passion, will frequently retreat from the rest of the world and spend a good deal of time on sex, food and calling in sick. Unfortunately, even conscientious dieters, their appetites stimulated by love, tend toward rich, sensual foods, and unless there is compensatory sexual activity, baby fat will almost certainly begin to appear.

Comparison of Foods Eaten When:

Not in love	In love
Tuna on rye	Pâté on French bread
Yogurt	Ice cream
Carrots	Halvah
Tangerine	Blueberries in whipped cream
English muffin	Griddle cakes and sausage
Mineral water	Wine
Porridge	Caviar
Antibiotics	Chocolate
Hard-boiled egg	Quiche
Wheat germ	Fried chicken
Licking lips	Licking partner's lips

Symptoms of Love

When are you officially in love? The symptoms are so varied that many people, even trained paramedics, confuse being in love with everything from tropical disease to temporary sanity. Here, however, are some reliable signs.

Activity	Calories burned
Walking on air	85
Walking on water	379
Dissolving	500
Feeling ten feet tall	62
Hitting your head	90
Sending flowers	14
Collect	45
Phoning more than five times a day	31
Phoning more than five times an hour	93
Dialing	13
Touch-toning	6½
Grinning	23
Glowing	17
In the dark	59

Intimacy

Letting down your defenses, showing you're vulnerable—admitting that you faint at the sight of milk or that a really fluffy wash can make you shed tears — isn't that what it's really all about?

Activity	Calories burned
Admitting that you wear	
A toupee	31
Contact lenses	17
Contact paper	55
Elevator shoes	45
False fingernails	18
False fingertips	95
Confessing that you had	
Nose job: bump removed	28
bump inserted	80
Face-lift	69
Face-hoist	100
Revealing a passion for	
Junk food	30
Straight sugar cane	47
Music in elevators	54
Music only in elevators	75

Keeping a Woman Warm

It is in the fall that many women, rather than fight the cold alone, undergo a process known as "winterizing," in which they trade a thin, hairless lover for a larger, bearlike model, preferably one who is able to generate heat, much like a wood-burning stove or a well-chosen Yule log. The object, of course, is to prevent frostbite and shivering during long winter walks and sleeping in a heat-starved apartment.

Fortunately for the dieting male, being a heat object has its rewards. According to the Women's Council on Warmth, keeping the average woman warm requires a heat output that would "shame the surface of the sun." The process itself, termed "heat transfer," is simple but effective. While sleeping, the two partners cling together, and the calories relinquished by the male actually penetrate and enter the woman's skin and seep into her soul, thereby warming the cockles of her heart. Not only does this keep the woman warm, but it may also, unless she's still shivering, cause her to pick up a teeny amount of weight. The man, on the other hand, may find himself slightly lighter in the morning, thus explaining why large men prefer a hearty breakfast of scrambled eggs, potato pancakes and stout.

Activity	Calories burned by male
Snuggling	25
Hugging	34
Cuddling	40
Sex	
If woman participates	85
If she doesn't	179

If woman is petite 284
  Will require the most calories because few tiny
  women have a heat-producing apparatus of their own.

If woman is regular size 196
  This figure holds true unless she uses a thermal
  nightie. Then deduct twenty calories.

If woman is large 105
  Will also need heat but not as much. Man can even
  relax his hugging during the night without getting
  yelled at.

If woman is abundant . . . . −14
  Here, the system of heat transfer works in reverse:
  It is the male who is kept warm.

Really Getting It Together

Marriage

(For those wishing to experiment or who happen to get carried away.)

Activity	Calories burned
Marrying for	
Escape	210
Love	31
Money	643
Both	5
Great cooking	12
Perfect bone structure	48
Citizenship	216
Steady sex	100
Unsteady sex	245
Change of tax status	51
A wedding	98
Marrying to get out of the house	145

The Wedding Night

(For those who get married and *have a wedding night.)*

Activity	Calories burned
Carrying spouse over threshold	52
If spouse ate too much wedding cake	125
Making the first move	
If you are shy	27
If you forgot the sex manual	158
If photographer still taking pictures	200
Performance anxiety due to	
Cultural difference (spouse from Arkansas)	45
Conflicting astrological signs	18
Mother-in-law coaching	133
Spouse still opening gifts	251
Foreplay	60
No play	1
Doing it for the first time	
One partner experienced	78
Both partners experienced	149
Both partners inexperienced	657
Doing it for the second time	100
If both partners still inexperienced	800

Sex

Activity	Calories burned
Premarital sex	342
Postmarital sex	84

Maintaining Passion

(How to keep your love life from growing stale.)

Activity	Calories burned
Stop watching the clock.	49
Changing the night ordinarily reserved for sex	36
Changing the sheet ordinarily reserved for sex	17
Changing your approach	23
From north to south	58

Wearing unusual clothing
    Black nylon galoshes. 27
    Black lace knapsack 40
    Quilted loincloth 51

Spontaneous sex
    While doing the dishes. 39
    While repotting a fern 48
    On an exit ramp. 232

Affairs

An affair is a great calorie burner not only because of the intemperate quality of sex, but because of the complications—when and where to meet, trying not to be seen, suddenly running into old friends (469 calories—more if the old friend happens to be your spouse) and constantly inventing ingenious excuses.

Activity	Calories burned per encounter
Regular affair	
Male	175
Female	163
Older man, younger woman	
Male	92
Female	237
Older woman, younger man	
Female	574
Male	10
Much older woman, really old man	
Female	6
Male	3½
Professor and coed	
Professor	148
Coed: if doing it for love	190
if doing it for grades	366

Romantic Moments

Activity	Calories burned

A quiet evening at home
    Alone 27
    With a friend 45
    Who also happens to be your lover 79
    And a terrific lover at that 255

A not-so-quiet afternoon at a motel 500

Any shipboard romance
    With a complete stranger 143
    With an incomplete stranger 306

Communicating

In the beginning of a relationship, talking to each other may burn up more than 200 calories a day, even more if either party is slightly deaf. As the relationship progresses, however, conversation usually diminishes and, by the eighth month, communication may either cease altogether or else take the form of grunts, gestures and, during jocular moments, ideograms.

Activity	Calories burned
First hour of first date, when trying to establish a rapport	55
Second hour of first date, when trying to talk partner into bed	90
Tenth date, when trying to talk partner out of bed and to a movie or at least out to dinner	61
After four months of living together	38
After one year	10

Saying "I Love You"

Activity	Calories burned
To your partner	
Just before orgasm	3
Just after orgasm.	40
To yourself	2
To your dog.	8
To your psychiatrist	23
To a perfect cheeseburger	½

Saying "I Love It"

Activity	Calories burned
During sex.	¼

Jealousy

Feelings of jealousy, which can burn more calories than an uphill slalom, are usually aroused when one lover discovers trace elements (real or imagined) of a rival. The result can range anywhere from vague mental discomfort (62 calories) to a passionate rage during which you redo your lover's apartment with a flame thrower (933 calories).

Activity   **Calories burned**

Jealousy aroused by partner's:
    Sudden increase in business dinners 45
        (*more than six per week*)
    New, oddly youthful appearance, including
        bounce in step and abundant vim 53
    Excessive generosity toward you 60
        (*a new dune buggy, for instance*)
    Change of hairstyle 31
    Change of cologne. 75
    Change of underwear 145
    Taking a phone call in the next room 48
    Making a phone call in the next room. 90
    Sudden weight loss 81
    New exercise class 66
    Suspicious behavior—such as wearing
        dark glasses and a hat to bed 200
    Flirting at a dinner party: with an attractive guest 55
                               with an attractive roast. 10

Jealousy (results of)

Activity	Calories burned
Investigating partner's drawers and closets.	31
Feeling guilty	67
But feeling justified	80

Discovering love letters	
Yours	3
Not yours	318

Making certain to put things back exactly the way you found them	40
Not quite remembering how you found them.	100

Outrageous behavior	
Constantly sniffing partner	25
Dusting partner for strange fingerprints	53
Without letting partner know.	481

Quarrels

Activity	Calories burned
Tiff	3
Spat	5
Squabble	10
With refined name-calling	17
Stamping feet	20
Stamping partner's feet	35

Dueling
    Ladle versus ski pole 68
    Pencils at ten paces 7

Minor altercation (throwing dishes) 42
Major altercation (when they're full) 65

Not speaking to each other 1

Guerrilla tactics
    Glue in toothpaste 12
    Short-sheeting bed 15
    Hiding bathroom tissue 9
    No sex 20
    Some sex, but not of high quality 38

Warfare

Activity	Calories burned
Arguing over money	
Too much	3
Too little	258
Arguing over sex	
Too little	258
Too much	3

Making Up

Half the fun of arguing is making up. The other half is getting the furniture repaired.

Activity	Calories burned

Speaking first
    If argument your fault 47
    If argument your partner's fault 15

Apologizing
    If you're sincere 20
    If you're not 1

Fighting over who should apologize. 56

Resisting attempts to kiss and make up
    If partner naked 35
    And you're aroused. 90

Breaking Up

Sometimes things just don't work out.

Activity	Calories burned
Hiring a lawyer	62

Dividing possessions	
Books	34
Records	42
Clothing	75
A loaf of bread	6
The wind chimes	20
The dog (including visitation rights)	29

Working out plant custody	53

Returning keys	200

Deciding who moves out	
Tossing a coin	8
Arm wrestling	27
Going to court	453

Aftermath

"The first night is the hardest. Then, for the next few weeks, it gets worse."

Activity	Calories burned
Moping	4
Moping around	11
Feeling as though today is the last day of the rest of your life	23
Depression (*undereating*)	34
Extreme depression (*calling old lovers*)	45
Resolving to be strong	7
Being strong	215
Getting person out of your mind	3
Keeping person out of your mind	468
Resisting urge to call	1,000
Heartbreak Of loneliness	84
Of psoriasis	516

Falling Out of Love

Activity	Calories burned
Eating your heart out........................	14 (per bite)

Contact

Activity	Calories burned
Just being good friends	52
If you're still sexually attracted	790

The New You

Don't sit around feeling sorry for yourself. This burns a minimal number of calories and greatly reduces your chances of finding someone new.

Activity	Calories burned
Night school (per class)	214
Cruising bars (per bar)	408
Per rejection	45
Disco roller-skating	690
Disco skiing	982
Stamp collecting	54
Glass blowing	67
Glass sucking	518
Directing your feet to the sunny side of the street	100
Abstinence	
Voluntary	2
Involuntary	370

Finding a New Partner

Aside from parties, singles' bars, a house-to-house search and being in the right museum at the right time, one of the most effective ways to meet that special someone is an ad in your local newspaper. As you will see when the replies start pouring in, it is reassuring to be surrounded by a mountain of letters, all promising dates galore, several romantic encounters and a perfect life.

Activity	**Calories burned**
Composing the ad	
One that reflects the real you	28
One that will get responses	79
Describing yourself	
Accurately	14
Enticingly	53

A successful personal ad should be accurate, but not too accurate —this is no time to be modest. When describing yourself, make the most of your assets by combining imagination with fact. For further assistance, see the Asset Conversion Table on the following pages.

Asset Conversion Table

The real you:	How to word your ad:
An embarrassment to your parents.	Oddly spacy, yet strangely amusing, interested in tarot, metaphysics and Swedish movies.
Marginally attractive, annual cosmetics bill only slightly less than first-class jet fare to Malta.	Showgirl type.
Neurotic, high-strung, manipulative and domineering, have no idea what I want but hate to be alone.	Spirited individual, unafraid to sample the unknown, seeks warm, lasting relationship.
Convicted killer.	Lonely inmate.
Desperately unrealistic, forty-three years old, still trying to make the leap from shoe clerk to celluloid idol.	Hopeless romantic.
Tense, driven, plagued by mood swings and gamma rays. Only hope is astrology and a rogue pharmacist.	Zany, live-wire Virgo, no objection to taking a chance on life's Divine Comedy.
Still-joined, but very together Siamese twins.	Fantastic 2 for 1 offer.
Unblemished record of compulsive dependency. Spent last relationship under martial law.	Trusting individual, willing to give and give to someone who will take and take.

The real you:	How to word your ad:
Illegal alien seeking green card.	Sensuous newcomer to these shores. Object: matrimony and partnership in a hot dog wagon.
Overweight, out of shape, high heart attack risk.	Abundantly shapely and very huggable, great for cold-night cuddling.
Rigid, fearful of sexual contact.	So secure, will take no for an answer.
Raving drag queen	Connoisseur of vivid fabric.
In perfect health but only passable looks.	Beautiful on the inside, attractive on the outside.
No stranger to tranquilizers, would like to stay in bed forever, needs sedation before using public transportation.	Shy, sensitive, soul-of-a-poet; turned off by hustle-bustle, glittery type of life.
4'11", 84 pounds, obsessed with plants.	Petite nature lover.
Phone hasn't rung in four months.	Fed up with dull relationships.

Note: If you're responding to a personal ad, simply reverse the tables above. The person who wrote, "Bubbly, scintillating kook," may actually be an "Emotionally shredded outpatient, tired of wearing paper slippers."

Selecting Replies

Activity	Calories burned
With caution	27
With extreme caution (to avoid misfits)	95

A word of warning before making an assignation: As you will see below, there may be a slight discrepancy between what you advertised for and what you get—imagination works both ways.

What you said you want:	What you may get:
A very special person.	A Martian.
Multifaceted individual, in touch with needs, searching for excitement.	Born-again lunatic with lots of annoying habits, looking to overthrow the government.
Convivial madcap for delirious fun, carefree afternoons, merry evenings.	A problem drinker.
Good-looking adventurer with insatiable lust for life.	On-the-lam Corsican, heavily into the loan sharks.
Buxom tigress seeking amorous afternoons.	Overweight nympho, demands include a whipping at teatime.
Emotionally mature professional, ready to explore ecstasies of Venus.	Monotonous astronomer.

What you said you want:	What you may get:
Committed relationship.	A patient from the local asylum.
Meaningless sex with shallow, but perky all-American.	Failed majorette.
Lover to whom friendship, honesty and sincerity more important than sex.	Impotent religious fanatic.
Someone who is tired of dining alone.	A freeloader.
Kindred spirit.	Your cousin.
Conservative, even-tempered companion for quiet evenings in front of a fire.	Lassie.

VII. Even More Sex

Because, for so many people, life proceeds from coitus to inter-ruptus, we felt it necessary to offer the dieter yet another means of losing weight without rushing out and buying a sauna.

Sexual activity has long been considered to be an excellent way to shed pounds. Not only is it efficient, it's also cheap (no expensive lessons or waiting for a court), pleasurable and, unless you've chosen an exceptionally selfish partner,* there are no feelings of deprivation.

In *The Dieter's Guide to Weight Loss During Sex,* it was pointed out that, at sea level, the average sex act consumes 350 calories, and the above-average sex act nearly 14,721 (between two psychotic elephants, for example). Over the past year, how-ever, new developments in modern technology and partners have shed new light on what occurs, calorically, during sexual activity, including a revealing look at the causal connection be-tween a particularly satisfying orgasm and the demolition of baby fat.†

This, and an abundance of additional weight loss information will be found on the following pages.

*See Chapter II, "Rolling Over and Going to Sleep."
†Not to mention teenage fat and adult fat.

What Is Sex?

Since, in this chapter, we are dealing with sex as an instrument of weight loss (with a little pleasure thrown in), we will define sex as any act of intimacy that generates moisture. Perhaps, though, we should also ask, why is sex? And what, besides weight loss, are the reasons for having it? Sexual motivation falls into five broad categories, each of which burns calories accordingly.

Reason for sex	Calories burned

Desire 312

The most popular form of sex, one that ends with a whimper and begins with a bang. Symptoms include a zooming heart rate and prolonged moaning. At its most extreme, partners may engage in sexual rites not yet sanctioned by the United Nations.

Remedial 250

Principal motivation here is weight loss, ego restoration and general shape-up—chasing stray cellulites and achieving a yummier behind. Because of its calming effect, remedial sex makes a perfect relaxant before, after and during hang-gliding.

Humanitarian 124

Here, sex is administered out of generosity—in tribute to one's partner or to improve the welfare of another, often with utter indifference to one's own pleasure and well-being. The sexual humanitarian will also give aid to the sexually deprived, such as a sailor with ten minutes' shore leave. Typical humanitarian may, with every orgasm, throw in a free set of drinking glasses.

Sex used in lieu of cash—to pay one's share of dinner, a contribution to your favorite charity or to repay a favor such as smuggling a couch across the border. Also in this category: Satisfying a partner who is in the mood when you're not and test-driving a new sex manual. Few significant weight loss benefits in this category.

To fend off boredom when there's nothing on television and to compensate for inclement weather on your honeymoon. Also a good diversion while driving across Texas.

Are You Sexually Rigid?

The ability to perform at a moment's notice, do it with an Albanian and cope with sex no matter what the season will greatly influence your weight loss program.

- Are you always orgasmic or are you thrown by the smell of Aqua Velva?
- Can you adjust to a new partner's pace (say a jazz drummer) or must you always set the rhythm?
- During intercourse, are you lost without a metronome?
- If necessary, could you change your clothes in the rear of a speeding taxi? And get your eyelashes on straight?
- Would you still have sex even if you knew for sure you were not going to lose weight?
- Can you drink red wine with a fishy partner?
- Would you be put off by a partner with a Q-shaped organ?
- Would you give up sex if they found it caused gout in laboratory mice?
- After sex, have you ever been tempted to nibble the sheet?
- What is the highest level of education you have completed?

Preparing for Sex

Activity	Calories burned

Taping wrists 15

Taking phone off the hook 3

Dusting off your erogenous zones 26

Memorizing partner's name 12
Jotting it on the ceiling 21

Aphrodisiacs
    Bark of yohimbé tree (per bite) 5
    M&M's (per M) 3
    Geritol 9

Flipping the sheets 18

Dimming the lights 4
By blowing out the bulbs 268

Showing stag film 15
With real stags 50

All-purpose mood music
    "Thirty Unforgettable Hawaiian Hits" 102
    "Thirty Forgettable Hawaiian Hits" 102

Typing thank-you note 10

Encouraging partner to lie down 6

If partner not tired. 63

Things Often Said Before Sex

Activity	Calories burned
Any sexually related utterance 8	

Examples
     "Put your knitting down."
     "Have a vitamin."
     "Your bed or mine?"
     "You drive, I'm sleepy."
     "Will I still have to take the final?"
     "Race you to the bed."
     "I want you to be the mother of my children."
     "Fill 'er up."

Initiating Sexual Activity

Activity	Calories burned
Flirting	6
Putting down your fork	2
Giving secret signal	5
Panting	3
Taking off glasses	4
Food fight	64
Scrawling message on mirror	9
If partner doesn't get message	25
If partner doesn't want to get message	62

Obstacles to Perfect Sex

Excuses	Calories burned

Might wake the children 23
Might wake the dog 68
Might wake me 195

Neighbors might hear 30
And get envious 49

Only sleeping permitted at this motel 91

Ache
      Back 15
      Tooth 12
      Head 18
      None of the above 57

Mudpack solidified 74
Hairdo too voluminous 80
Sunburn 25

Not properly sedated 66

Okay, but no physical contact 100

Still working hours 49
Desk too small 67

Watching important cartoon 30

No appointment 46

We just did it last week 59

Persuasion

Activity	Calories burned
Asking nicely	19
Wheedling	28
Coaxing	37
Pleading	46
Begging	53
Bribing	
New couch	65
Swearing not to bother partner	
for another two months	92

Saying "Yes"

Reasons	Calories burned

To lose weight. 5

To improve complexion. 11

Out of curiosity
    New partner. 15
    New activity. 48

Because
    You want to. 1
    Your partner wants you to. 26
    It's the only way you'll get a lift home 60

Saying "No"

Reasons	Calories burned
You don't want to	14
You've lost enough weight.	4
You need more time to think	23
You really mean yes	1
If partner takes you seriously	75
Parents would not approve	48
Uncertain of partner's sexual identity (*bar too dark*)	67
Uncertain of partner's sexual preference.	97
Shabby underwear	143

Undressing for Sex

When should clothing be removed? To facilitate physical contact, clothing should be discarded well before the fifth kiss. If outdoors, even sooner to avoid grass stains. Some feel, however, that it is more natural to undress gradually. This has its drawbacks: the temptation not to fold one's clothes neatly, thereby increasing the danger of unsightly wrinkles. And finally, once your partner is undressed there may be a few surprises.

Activity	Calories burned
Partner too big for his britches	39
Partner too big for your britches	53
Reacting to partner's endowment	
If average endowment	24
If small and unassuming	10
If un-average endowment (twelve inches, relaxed)	458
Marvelling	29
Cheering	41
Pretending not to notice	63
Undoing partner's bra	
Regular	7
With combination lock	55

Dressing for Sex

Wearing	Calories burned
Sweat bands	8
Spurs	25
That jingle	33
Roll-on musk oil	10
Roll-in musk oil	54
Wet suit made in Hong Kong	28
Bondage girdle	23
With plunging neckline	50
Totes	15
G-string	9
Truss	17
With back pocket	21
Strait jacket	36
With lapels	54

Telling Partner What Gets You Excited

Activity	Calories burned

Level I 15

Pretty much the usual—your basic hugging, kissing, standard foreplay and nothing more adventurous than massaging the sex manual with baby oil.

Level II... 27

A bit out of the ordinary. May involve an artificial erotic device powered by batteries.

Level III 68

Make certain you know your partner well. Covers any intimacy utilizing lotion or exotic rubber attire such as a wide-belted radial. May also include talking on the phone to your parents during foreplay. (Add ten calories if you let your partner say hello.)

If you're shy and can't discuss sex

Suffering in silence 90

Just leaving a note on the windshield 24

Arousal

Activity	Calories burned

Kissing
    French (with tongue in mouth) 14
    English (with cigarette in mouth). 28
    American (with pizza in mouth) 40

Nibbling 12

Biting 19

Teething.. 14

Just gumming it a little. 5

Making partner tingle
    With lips 25
    With wall socket 112

Blowing in partner's ear
    Taking aim 6
    Missing.. 11
    Arousing dog, instead 60

Gourmet wrestling 92

What Else Arouses You?

Activity	Calories burned
Indoor plumbing	12
Inner plumbing	50
Partner dressed in leather	30
Partner dressed in Ultra-suede	6
Partner wearing housedress	
Yours	21
His	45
Group sex	
You, your partner and a friend	58
You, a celebrity animal and its trainer	66
You and a conglomerate	93
Finding a new erogenous zone	27
Rediscovering an old one	38
Slow, lingering foreplay	41
Free tickets to a sporting event	57
Getting searched	32
By partner named Dr. Strange-Glove	100

Foreplay

Activity	Calories burned
Normal night	76
Bowling night	4

When Is It Time?

Activity	Calories burned
Partner ticking	17
Glasses fogging up	20
Face fogging up	46
Ready to stop the car	33
Telltale glow	21
Mineral oil bubbling	40
Religious medal overheating	97

Taking Precautions

Activity   **Calories burned**

Using
    Latex contraceptive 11
       If warranty fails 298
    Designer version with raised lettering. 63
    Lambskin 8
    Fishskin 12
    Asbestos. 367
       (prevents overheating)
    Any whimsical device 28
       (with a face and little ears)
    Saran Wrap. 19
       (to keep it fresh)

Unwrapping contraceptive
    Well beforehand 5
    In the heat of passion. 78
    While trying to read the instructions 92
    Which are in Danish. 137

Putting it on
    With erection 3
    Without erection. 258
    Without removing foil 500

Inserting diaphragm 9
During intercourse 311

Intercourse

Activity	Calories burned
Striking while the iron is hot	128
Striking while the iron is not so hot	5

Insertion	3
While negotiating a hairpin turn	259

Best positions for spot reducing*
　　Upper thighs: you on bottom, partner on top 28
　　Upper arms: partner on bottom, you doing push-ups. . . . 45
　　Stomach: partner on top, you doing sit-ups 57
　　Upper abdomen: partner on bottom, you doing
　　　　sit-downs 62
　　Lower abdomen: standing face to face 52
　　Hips: standing up, back to back 449

Spot enlarging 70
　　(indicates you're doing something right)

*Greasing the sheets will cut your turnaround time in half.

Orgasm

Activity	Calories burned
For woman	
Vaginal	27
Clitoral	31
A blend	40
Can't tell	65

For man	
Regular ejaculation (honorable discharge)	35
Premature ejaculation (dishonorable discharge): while still mixing drinks	3
while asking for a date	½

Simultaneous orgasm	56
If earth moves	90
If only building moves	23
If partner moves	126

Self-Defense

In case partner is going for a record but you want to (or have to) stop.

Activity	Calories burned
Faking orgasm	64
Faking sleep . . . . :	82
Faking asthma	
Air quality good	78
Air quality poor	5

How to Calculate Multiple Orgasm Table

	1	2	3	4	5	6	7	8	9
1	1	2	3	4	5	6	7	8	9
2	2	4	6	8	10	12	14	16	18
3	3	6	9	12	15	18	21	24	27
4	4	8	12	16	20	24	28	32	36
5	5	10	15	20	25	30	35	40	45
6	6	12	18	24	30	36	42	48	54
7	7	14	21	28	35	42	49	56	63
8	8	16	24	32	40	48	56	64	72
9	9	18	27	36	45	54	63	72	81

Side Effects of Multiple Orgasm

Activity	Calories burned
Losing count	7
One-inch grin	20
Two-inch grin	32
Six-inch grin	50
Twinkle in eye	23
Twinkle in both eyes	46
Babbling	68
But making sense	90
Putting partner out to pasture	117

Front Effect of Multiple Orgasm

Activity	Calories burned
Moisture.	10

Weight Loss Bonus #2

Activity	Calories burned
Not avoiding the wet spot	18
If it's well-chilled	144

Spontaneous Sex

Activity	Calories burned

On an elevator 61
With bouncy music 88
With bouncy passengers 196

In the kitchen
    While basting a roast 49
    While basting a partner 75
    While dinner guests waiting. 31
    Between courses 19

On a picnic 50
With an innerspring blanket. 67
With ants 274

In a plane
    During the movie 52
    If flight attendant keeps pestering you 98
    For more sex 124
    Orgasm while landing 60
    Bonus orgasm: finding your luggage 115

At the office 53
After 5:00 P.M. 65
Putting in for supper money 14

Under water 39
While diving for treasure 56

Things Often Said After Sex

Activity	Calories burned
Any utterance...............................	10

Examples
    "S.O.S."
    "Love your hair."
    "That was my first time."
    "That was my last time."
    "Help me breathe."
    "Mind if I light up?"
    "This time using a match?"
    "Your orgasm or mine?"
    "King me!"
    "Okay, start the elevator."
    "Coffee!"
    "I can't fine-tune my eyes."
    "Is anything missing."

Things Often Said
Way After Sex

Activity	Calories burned
"I've got something to tell you."	358
"I've got something to show you."	1,000

Light Housekeeping

Activity	Calories burned
Closing sex manual 2	
Returning it to shelf. 11	
Returning it to library 46	
Paying overdue fine 3	
Paying damage fine 10	